Breast Cancer / Bosom Malignant growth

Kick breast cancer out of your life, reclaim your healthy lifestyle, and never experience breast cancer again for the rest of your life.

By

Kathy B. Kehoe

Disclaimer

On the off chance that you buy this book without a cover or buy a PDF, JPG, or spat duplicate of it, it is marvelously taken property or a fake. Considering everything, neither the creators, the vendor, nor any of their workers or specialists have gotten any piece of the duplicate. Furthermore, ravaging is a known road to monetary help for workers with terrible ways to deal with acting and mental attacker parties. We demand that you not buy any such duplicates and report any occasion of somebody offering such duplicates to Plata Appropriating LLC.

This scattering is expected to give skilled and solid data concerning the subject covered. At any rate, is sold with the appreciation that the creator and merchant have not participated in conveying good 'old-fashioned, cash-related, or another expert course. Rules and practices on occasion change beginning with one state and afterward going and country to country, and expecting valid or other master help is required, the relationship of an expert ought to be looked for.

The writer and dealer unequivocally deny any obligation that is achieved by the usage or use of the things in this book.

Introducing

At any point do you accept that individuals kicked the bucket since they have Bosom Disease? All that you catch wind of bosom disease is completely false.

Certain individuals do accept that disease spells almost certain doom for the street, yet it's not the very thing you think.

Malignant growth can be a hazardous infection yet it doesn't mean it will kill you.

Hi everybody! I go by **Kathy B. Kehoe,** I'm an individual of 62 years of age from Dallas.

I was a specialist in an emergency clinic in Plano when I was 29 years of age, I had the bosom disease and I was unable to treat it at my medical clinic, and this made me think I planned to bite the dust, I went through a few medical procedures and there was no solution for malignant growth, I began living in dread and torment believe that is the stopping point for me. On one occasion I met a lady in Arlington who was a bosom malignant growth subject matter expert, following fourteen days of therapy I got from him, I recuperated from bosom disease and became solid and sound till this exact second I'm very well sound.

After I recuperated from bosom malignant growth, I chose to begin working with her, and I worked with her for an additional 32 years.

Dear peruser! The items in this book are rigorously to tell you how to forestall bosom disease and how to be aware assuming you are creating bosom malignant growth side effects at a beginning phase.

The items in this book are precisely the things I have encountered, learned, and shown individuals who created bosom malignant growth around me and it has turned out great for them. I chose to compose this book in other to connect with additional individuals out there and save additional individuals from bosom malignant growth sickness. Individuals have been giving declarations and my educating and you can likewise be a piece of them by getting yourself a duplicate of this book. Remain Favored.

Table of contents

Part One

What is Breast Cancer/ Bosom Malignant growth

Bosom malignant growth is a sickness where cells in the bosom outgrow control. There are several types of breast cancer. The sort of breast cancer relies upon which cells in the breast transform into disease.

Most bosom tumors start in the pipes or lobules. The bosom disease can spread externally the bosom through veins and lymph vessels. In the area where breast cancer grows to several pieces of the body, it is said to have metastasized.

Sorts of Bosom Disease

The most well-known sorts of bosom disease are:
Obtrusive ductal carcinoma. The disease cells start in the channels and afterward develop outside the conduits into different pieces of the bosom tissue.

Obtrusive malignant growth cells can likewise spread, or metastasize, to different pieces of the body.

Obtrusive lobular carcinoma. Malignant growth cells start in the lobules and afterward spread from the lobules to the bosom tissues that are nearby. These obtrusive disease cells can likewise spread to different pieces of the body.

The areola is the opening in the skin of the bosom where the pipes meet up and transform into bigger conduits so the milk can leave the bosom. The areola is encircled by marginally more obscure thicker skin called the areola. A more uncommon sort of bosom malignant growth called Paget illness of the bosom can begin in the areola.

The fat and connective tissue (stroma) encompass the pipes and lobules and assist with keeping them set up. A more uncommon kind of bosom disease called phyllodes growth can begin in the stroma.

Veins and lymph vessels are discovered in each bosom. Angiosarcoma is a more uncommon sort of bosom disease that can begin in the covering of these vessels.

How bosom malignant growth spreads

Bosom malignant growth can spread when the disease cells get into the blood or lymph framework and afterward are conveyed to different pieces of the body.

The lymph (or lymphatic) framework is a piece of your body's invulnerable framework. It is an organization of lymph hubs (little, bean-sized organs), pipes or vessels, and organs that cooperate to gather and help clear lymph liquid through the body tissues to the blood. The unmistakable lymph liquid inside the lymph vessels contains tissue results and waste material, as well as invulnerable framework cells.

The lymph vessels divert lymph liquid from the bosom. On account of bosom disease, disease cells can enter those lymph vessels and begin to fill in lymph hubs. The vast majority of the lymph vessels of the bosom channel into:

Lymph hubs under the arm (axillary lymph hubs)

Lymph hubs inside the chest close to the breastbone (interior mammary lymph hubs)

Lymph hubs around the collar bone (supraclavicular [above the collar bone] and infraclavicular [below the collar bone] lymph hubs)

Assuming malignant growth cells have spread to your lymph hubs, there is a higher opportunity that the cells might have gone through the lymph framework and spread (metastasized) to different pieces of your body. In any case, not all ladies with malignant growth cells in their lymph hubs foster metastases, and a few ladies with no disease cells in their lymph hubs could foster metastases later.

What causes bosom malignant growth?

Bosom disease happens when there are changes in the hereditary material (DNA). Frequently, the specific reason for these hereditary changes is obscure.

However, some of the time these hereditary changes are acquired, implying that you are brought into the world with them.

A bosom disease that is brought about by acquired hereditary changes is called genetic bosom malignant growth.

There are additionally certain hereditary changes that can raise your gamble of bosom disease, remembering changes for the BRCA1 and BRCA2 qualities. These two changes likewise raise your gamble of ovarian and other diseases.

Other than hereditary qualities, your way of life and the climate can influence your gamble of bosom disease.

Who is in danger of bosom disease?

The elements that raise your gamble of bosom malignant growth include:

More seasoned age

History of bosom malignant growth or harmless (noncancer) bosom illness

Acquired hazard of bosom malignant growth, including having BRCA1 and BRCA2 quality changes

Thick bosom tissue

A regenerative history that prompts more openness to the estrogen chemical, including

Bleeding at an early age

Being at a more seasoned age when you previously conceived an offspring or never having conceived an offspring

Beginning menopause at a later age

Taking chemical treatment for side effects of menopause

Radiation treatment to the bosom or chest

Weight

Drinking liquor

Will bosom malignant growth be forestalled?

You might have the option to assist with forestalling bosom malignant growth by making solid way-of-life changes, for example,

Remaining at a solid weight

Restricting liquor use

Getting enough exercise

Restricting your openness to estrogen by

Breastfeeding your infants if possible

Restricting chemical treatment

Assuming you are at a high gamble, your medical care supplier might recommend that you take specific drugs to bring down the gamble. A few ladies at exceptionally high gamble might choose to get a mastectomy (of their solid bosoms) to forestall bosom malignant growth.

Getting ordinary mammograms is likewise significant. They might have the option to distinguish bosom malignant growth in the beginning phases when it is more straightforward to treat.

Part Two

Dcis bosom disease

DCIS is an early bosom disease. It implies that a few cells in the coating of the conduits of the bosom tissue have begun to transform into malignant growth cells. These cells are contained inside the pipes. They have not begun to spread into the encompassing bosom tissue.

Ductal carcinoma in situ (DCIS) is the presence of strange cells inside a milk conduit in the bosom.
DCIS is viewed as the earliest type of bosom malignant growth. DCIS is painless, meaning it hasn't fanned out of the milk pipe and is generally safe from becoming obtrusive.
DCIS is typically found during a mammogram done as a feature of bosom disease screening or to research a bosom knot.
While DCIS isn't a crisis, it requires an assessment and a thought of treatment choices. Therapy might incorporate bosom monitoring a medical procedure

joined with radiation or a medical procedure to eliminate all of the bosom tissue. A clinical preliminary concentrating on dynamic observing as an option in contrast to a medical procedure might be another choice.

Ductal carcinoma in situ (DCIS) is a condition that can happen in a few distinct structures. In these, there's an adjustment of the cells coating the milk channels of the bosom. Under a magnifying lens, an ordinary pipe shows a covering of a solitary layer of cells, yet in DCIS, a lot more cells should be visible. Frequently the cells nearly fill the pipe, as outlined underneath. For certain ladies, DCIS is tracked down in a couple of pipes, yet for other people, it very well might be found in a large part of the conduit arrangement of the bosom.

These additional cells in the conduit show a portion of the irregularities of disease cells, however haven't spread external the pipe (in that frame of mind 'set up'). Thus, DCIS isn't viewed as 'valid' or obtrusive malignant growth. At the point when left untreated, DCIS might advance and attack close-by bosom tissue, turning into a 'genuine' bosom disease.

Be that as it may, we can't anticipate whether or when this will happen, so the condition should be dealt with. Therapy for DCIS ought to have a generally excellent result since it ought to forestall movement to an intrusive bosom malignant growth

Causes

It's not satisfactory what causes DCIS. DCIS structures when hereditary changes happen in the DNA of bosom pipe cells. The hereditary transformations make the cells seem unusual, however, the cells don't yet break out of the bosom conduit.

Scientists don't know precisely the exact thing that triggers the unusual cell development that prompts DCIS. Factors that might have an impact incorporate your way of life, your current circumstances, and qualities passed to you from your folks.

Risk Elements

Factors that might expand your gamble on DCIS include:

Expanding age

The individual history of harmless bosom infection, like abnormal hyperplasia

Family background of bosom disease

Never having been pregnant

Having your most memorable child after the age of 30

Having your most memorable period before age 12

Starting menopause after age 55

Hereditary changes that increment the gamble of bosom malignant growth, like those in the bosom disease qualities BRCA1 and BRCA2

Finding and treatment of ductal carcinoma in situ

As screening mammography turns out to be more normal, DCIS is analyzed more frequently than previously. All the more seldom, a lady might be determined to have DCIS after she finds a bosom change, for example, a bump or an areola release.

DCIS can frequently be viewed as a specific example of little calcifications on the mammogram. Albeit the shape and size of the calcification might recommend DCIS to the radiologist, the finding should be affirmed by additional examination. The specialist will typically suggest a center needle biopsy, which includes the evacuation of a fragment of tissue through a needle under a nearby sedative. This tissue is then shipped off to a pathologist. The analysis may likewise be made by careful (open) biopsy. A careful biopsy is finished in a medical clinic, yet you typically will not need to remain for the time being.

Treatment for DCIS relies upon every lady's circumstance. More frequently than before, specialists can offer moderate treatment. This implies the specialist will just eliminate the area of DCIS, alongside a little line of unaffected tissue. Once in a while, further therapy by radiation will be recommended. Radiation treatment can have side impacts, and you ought to learn about these before beginning a course of therapy. See our Radiotherapy page for more.

After this moderate medical procedure is finished, regardless of radiation, there's some gamble of repeat. Once in a while, the repeat will be DCIS (still inside the pipe), however, at times it will be obtrusive bosom disease (spreading into the tissue outside the conduit). There's no proof of any advantage from axillary analyzation (expulsion of lymph hubs from the armpit) in ladies with DCIS 1.

For certain ladies, the specialist will suggest a mastectomy (evacuation of the impacted bosom). No further therapy is required for that bosom following mastectomy, and the future gamble of bosom malignant growth turns out to be tiny — around 1%. The other bosom ought to be consistently checked by mammography and actual assessment.

Ductal bosom malignant growth

Ductal bosom malignant growth starts in your milk channels. It incorporates obtrusive ductal carcinoma (IDC) and ductal carcinoma in situ (DCIS).

Ductal bosom malignant growth is the most well-known sort of bosom disease, and bosom malignant growth is the most widely recognized type of disease in the US.

Roughly 297,790 individuals in the US will get a bosom malignant growth finding in 2023. Given information from 2017 to 2019, around 13% of ladies will be determined to have female bosom disease during their lifetime.

Even though bosom disease regularly influences cisgender ladies and others relegated females upon entering the world, it's additionally feasible for individuals doled out males upon entering the world to foster bosom malignant growth.

Ductal bosom malignant growth makes up most instances of male bosom disease, as per the Habitats for Infectious Prevention (CDC)

Are there various kinds of ductal bosom disease?

There are two fundamental sorts:

Obtrusive ductal carcinoma (IDC): This kind of malignant growth makes up around 70-80% of all bosom diseases analyzed. It starts in the milk channels and spreads to the encompassing tissues.

Ductal carcinoma in situ (DCIS): DCIS is viewed as a beginning phase of malignant growth, harmless disease, or pre-malignant growth, as it hasn't yet begun to spread into the remainder of the bosom tissue. DCIS may ultimately prompt IDC.

What side effects are related to ductal bosom disease?

Side effects might include:

a little knot in the bosom

areola withdrawal

areola release that isn't bosom milk

peau d'orange (orange strip-like skin on your bosom)

determined bosom or areola torment

layered skin on your areola or bosom

skin disturbance

expanding of your bosom

thickening of the skin on your bosom

It means quite a bit to take note that the vast majority with ductal bosom disease experience no side effects. This is particularly valid for DCIS. Customary bosom malignant growth screenings can help identify ductal bosom disease in its beginning phases.

Most bosom side effects or changes aren't brought about by malignant growth. Yet, if you truly do see any surprising side effects, it's ideal to make a meeting with a medical care professional to check for unusual cells.

What causes ductal bosom malignant growth and who's most in danger?

Likewise, with different types of malignant growth, it's not clear why certain individuals create ductal bosom disease, and some don't.

Notwithstanding, specialists have distinguished that specific gatherings are bound to foster bosom disease more than others.

Risk factors for ductal bosom malignant growth include:

Progress in years: As you age, your gamble of creating bosom disease increases.

Liquor use: Regular drinking or liquor use jumble raises your gamble.

Certain conceptive elements: Individuals are bound to foster bosom disease on the off chance that they started bleeding before the age of 12, began menopause after 55, have never conveyed a pregnancy to term, or conceived an offspring at a more seasoned age.

Thick bosom tissue: Certain individuals normally have thick bosom tissue. This can build your gamble of bosom malignant growth and make mammograms harder to peruse.

Family background of bosom disease: You might be bound to foster bosom malignant growth on the off chance that a nearby female relative has had it. Be that as it may, the vast majority who foster it have no family background of the infection.

Qualities: On the off chance that you have specific quality changes, for example, BRCA1 and BRCA2, you're bound to foster bosom disease than individuals who don't.

History of bosom disease: On the off chance that you've had bosom malignant growth previously, you might foster it once more — perhaps in your other bosom or an alternate region of your bosom.

Chemical treatment: Postmenopausal estrogen and progesterone prescriptions might build your gamble of bosom disease. Transsexual ladies might be bound to foster bosom malignant growth more than cisgender men, potentially because of chemical treatment.

Smoking tobacco: There's a connection between smoking tobacco and bosom malignant growth. Openness to handed-down cigarette smoke may likewise build your gamble.

On the off chance that you figure you might be in danger of creating bosom disease, talk with a medical services professional. They can exhort you on how frequently you ought to get a mammogram too as a way of life transforms you can make to assist with decreasing your general gamble.

How is ductal bosom disease analyzed?

A medical care proficient will ordinarily play out a few tests to distinguish and analyze ductal bosom malignant growth.

This incorporates:

Actual test: Your PCP will physically analyze your bosom for protuberances or thickening.

Mammogram: A mammogram is an X-beam of your bosom that can identify malignant growth.

Biopsy: Your primary care physician will send an example of your bosom tissue to a lab to be inspected. A bosom biopsy can help decide whether a bump in your bosom is destructive or harmless.

Ultrasound: A bosom ultrasound utilizes sound waves to give a definite perspective on bosom tissue and bloodstream. It doesn't utilize radiation and is all right for individuals who are pregnant.

Attractive reverberation imaging (X-ray): X-rays can identify little bosom sores. Specialists use bosom X-rays to screen individuals with a high gamble of creating bosom disease.

The following stage is to decide the phase of the breast cancer:

Stage 0: There are strange cells in your conduits, however they aren't spreading yet. DCIS is viewed as stage 0.

Stage 1: The malignant growth is just in your bosom, with cancer 2 centimeters (cm) or 0.75 inches (in) or less in breadth.

Stage 2: The malignant growth has spread to local lymph hubs, or the cancer is 2-5 cm (0.75-2 in) in breadth.

Stage 3: The disease has spread widely in your bosom, encompassing tissues, and lymph hubs, yet all at once no further.

Stage 4: The disease has metastasized, meaning it's spread to additional far-off destinations in your body.

On the off chance that a medical care proficient has determined you to have DCIS, they might grade it. This evaluating framework is utilized to rate the probability of your DCIS returning after treatment:
High-grade, atomic grade 3, or high mitotic rate: DCIS has a higher probability of growing again after treatment.
Middle of the road level, atomic level 2, or halfway mitotic rate: DCIS is more averse to return after treatment.
Poor quality, atomic grade 1, or low mitotic rate: This grade of DCIS is to the least extent liable to return after treatment.

How is ductal bosom malignant growth treated?

An oncologist, a specialist who works in disease, will suggest a treatment plan given:
the kind of disease you have the stage and grade of the malignant growth your particular well-being needs

Ductal bosom malignant growth medicines include:

Medical procedure: This can incorporate a lumpectomy, which jams however much of your bosom as could be expected while eliminating the unusual cells and encompassing tissues, or a mastectomy, which eliminates however much bosom tissue as could reasonably be expected.

Radiation treatment: This treatment utilizes high-energy pillars to harm the DNA of strange and dangerous cells.

Hormonal treatment: Your clinician could recommend hormonal treatments on the off chance that disease cells are filling in light of estrogen and progesterone.

Chemotherapy: You as a rule wouldn't require chemotherapy for DCIS, however, it's frequently utilized for IDC after a lumpectomy or mastectomy. It can decrease the probability of disease spreading. Designated treatment: This therapy impedes the spread of atomic targets related to disease.

Immunotherapy: This treatment sets off your insusceptible framework to annihilate malignant growth cells.

What's the standpoint for somebody with ductal bosom malignant growth?

Your standpoint relies upon many variables, including the phase of determination.

The 5-year relative endurance rate for bosom malignant growth is around 90.8%. This is normal across all bosom malignant growth subtypes and stages.

Limited bosom malignant growth (that is, the disease hasn't spread past the bosom tissue) has a 99.3% 5-year relative endurance rate. The rate drops to 86.3% for regionalized bosom disease and 31% for bosom malignant growth that has spread to far-off pieces of the body.

DCIS, which is stage 0 ductal bosom malignant growth, has a 100 percent 5-year endurance rate. A recent report, which took a gander at 100,000 ladies north of 20 years, found that the main 3.3% percent of ladies treated for DCIS later kicked the bucket from bosom malignant growth.

The endurance rate for bosom disease has consistently expanded after some time, mostly given fresher and more compelling medicines.

Part Three

Icis bosom Malignant growth

Lobular carcinoma in situ (LCIS), otherwise called lobular neoplasia, is an uncommon condition where strange cells are fostered in the milk organs, known as lobules, in the bosom. These unusual cells are not viewed as a bosom disease and require no treatment past careful evacuation. In any case, the presence of LCIS might expand the patient's gamble of creating bosom disease in one or the other bosom from here on out. More forceful bosom disease screening or safeguard measures might be suggested.

Lobular carcinoma in situ (LCIS) implies that cells inside a portion of the bosom lobules have begun to become unusual. LCIS It's anything but a malignant growth.

The lobules are organs that make bosom milk. The strange cells are held inside the inward covering of the lobules. LCIS is additionally called lobular neoplasia. It very well may be tracked down in the two bosoms.

LCIS isn't a malignant growth, however having it implies that you have a little expanded chance of getting the obtrusive bosom disease in one or the other bosom from now on. All things being equal, most ladies with LCIS will not foster bosom malignant growth. Men can foster LCIS however this is exceptionally intriguing.

Lobular carcinoma in situ (LCIS) happens in the linings of milk-creating organs inside the bosom — the lobules. Albeit lobular carcinoma in situ contains "carcinoma" (one more name for the disease), it is not a type of bosom malignant growth. LCIS is a gamble factor, notwithstanding, for creating bosom disease later on. LCIS is a treatable condition and the viewpoint is great for the individuals who are determined to have it.

Bosom specialist Melissa Camp, M.D., M.P.H., makes sense of what you ought to be aware of lobular carcinoma in situ and how to function with your PCP to keep yourself protected and solid.

LCIS Side effects

Lobular carcinoma in situ doesn't as a rule cause side effects.

LCIS is regularly analyzed on a bosom biopsy performed for a strange mammogram and is just seen on a minute assessment of the bosom tissue. It is most regularly an accidental finding.

Analysis of Lobular Carcinoma in Situ LCIS might be determined to have a biopsy. A nearby glance at the LCIS cells by the pathologist can assist your PCP with settling on the subsequent stages of administration.

Bosom needle biopsy: "Lobular carcinoma in situ is typically determined to have a needle biopsy," Camp says. "The pathologist [a specialist who looks at body tissue for indications of disease] may recognize it unexpectedly when a biopsy is taken for another explanation."

After desensitizing the bosom region, a radiologist or specialist eliminates a modest quantity of bosom tissue by utilizing a needle. The example is shipped off a pathologist who takes a gander at the tissue under a magnifying lens and can affirm or preclude malignant growth cells.

"Now and again, the needle biopsy itself is adequate," Camp says. "At times, a marginally bigger example of the bosom tissue is expected to more conclusively preclude bosom disease, and a careful [excisional] bosom biopsy is performed."
Bosom excisional biopsy: "This is a minor strategy performed by a specialist to eliminate a somewhat bigger measure of bosom tissue where LCIS was distinguished," Camp makes sense of. "It often ends under broad sedation."

Whenever you are calm or snoozing, the specialist cuts the bosom and eliminates part or all of the area of concern. Now and again, the spot might be little, profound, and elusive, requiring the wire confinement strategy. For this, the radiologist or specialist embeds a needle with an extremely slim wire into the bosom and guides it into the area with LCIS utilizing X-beam pictures. With the wire set up, the specialist can recognize the region with LCIS and eliminate a tissue test for assessment under a magnifying lens.

Lobular Carcinoma in Situ Treatment

Checking and perception might be everything necessary. Camp tells patients determined to have LCIS not to overreact. "It just suggested that we have confessed that you might be at an upper gamble for generating bosom disease later on," she says.

"The main thing to do after determination," she adds, "is to find an extensive bosom community where your bosom wellbeing can be firmly checked and made due."

Camp underscores the significance of checking with imaging so that assuming bosom malignant growth is created, it very well may be recognized at the earliest conceivable stage. For patients with LCIS, we suggest yearly mammograms, and we may likewise propose yearly X-rays of the bosom for significantly nearer checking.

Furthermore, some drugs can assist with lessening the gamble of creating bosom disease later on. A conversation with your primary care physician about these meds can assist you with choosing if they are ideal for you.

Bosom a medical procedure may be a choice if you have other gamble factors for bosom malignant growth, like a BRCA quality change or other genetic component. Treatment can incorporate a preplanned (prophylactic) mastectomy.

What is the visualization for lobular carcinoma in situ?

Camp guarantees individuals determined to have LCIS that the visualization is awesome. With cautious checking with an accomplished specialist, patients with lobular carcinoma in situ have the most obvious opportunity to remain solid and disease-free.

Part Four

Vehicle immune system microorganism treatment

Bosom malignant growth ascends as the most usually analyzed disease in 2020. Among ladies, bosom disease positions first in both malignant growth occurrence rate and mortality.

Treatment obstruction created from the ongoing clinical treatments restricts the adequacy of restorative results, in this way new treatment approaches are direly required. Illusory antigen receptor (Vehicle) Lymphocyte treatment is a sort of immunotherapy created from supportive White blood cell movement, which ordinarily utilizes patients' insusceptible cells to battle disease.

Vehicle Lymphocytes are outfitted with explicit antibodies to perceive antigens in self-cancer cells consequently evoking cytotoxic impacts. As of late, Vehicle White blood cell treatment has accomplished amazing triumphs in treating hematologic malignancies; in any case, the restorative impacts in strong growths don't depend on assumptions including bosom disease. This survey means to examine the advancement of Vehicle White blood cell treatment in bosom disease from preclinical examinations to continuous clinical preliminaries.

In particular, we sum up growth-related antigens in bosom disease, continuous clinical preliminaries, hindrances obstructing the helpful impacts of Vehicle Lymphocyte treatment, and talk about possible procedures to further develop treatment viability.

By and large, we trust our survey gives a scene perspective on late advancement for Vehicle Immune system microorganism treatment in bosom malignant growth and lights interest for additional exploration bearings.

The worldwide disease measurements in 2020 show bosom malignant growth has superseded cellular breakdown in the lungs and become the most normally analyzed malignant growth around the world, with 2.3 million new cases in 11.7% of all disease types reported. Also, bosom malignant growth mortality positions fifth, with 685,000 patient passings in 20201. Among ladies, bosom malignant growth was analyzed in 1 of every 4 disease cases, and 1 out of 6 disease passing were brought about by bosom malignant growth, positioning the principal in both frequency rate and disease mortality1. The histological characterization of bosom disease is fundamentally founded on the articulation example of human epidermal development factor receptors 2 (HER2) and chemical receptors (HR) named estrogen receptors (emergency room) and progesterone receptors (PR), as well as the growth expansion rate showed by Ki-67, bringing about grouped 5 significant subtypes: HER2 positive, HR-positive (HER2+ and ER+ or PR+ or both positive); HER2 positive, HR negative (HER2+/trama center/PR-); basal-like or triple negative (HER2-/emergency room/PR-); luminal A (HER2-/ER+/PR+, low multiplication); and luminal B (HER2-/ER+/PR+, high proliferation)2.

The bosom malignant growth therapy is fundamental or nearby, given the bosom disease subtype and metastasis degree. For nonmetastatic bosom disease, the super remedial objectives are killing cancers from patients and forestalling growth repeat.

Nearby treatments including a medical procedure and radiation are utilized for growth destruction, while fundamental treatments comprising endocrine treatment, chemotherapy, and immunotherapy are utilized for additional destruction and repeat counteraction.

Foundational treatment might be neoadjuvant (preoperative), adjuvant (postoperative), or both. Bosom malignant growth subtypes guide the therapy draws near, for example, chemotherapy alone for triple-negative bosom disease, endocrine treatment for all HER2-/ER+/PR+ cancer, and immunotherapy (trastuzumab-based HER2-coordinated neutralizer) for all HER2+ cancer. For metastatic bosom disease, neighborhood treatment approaches alongside fundamental treatment approaches are commonly used to arrive at the primary treatment objectives of side effects lightening and dragging out life3.In many years, medical procedures, radiotherapy, chemotherapy, endocrine treatment, designated treatment, and immunotherapy have further developed the endurance rate and life nature of bosom malignant growth patients4, 5.

In any case, the mortality of bosom disease stays high to a great extent because of the reality that the created obstruction in patients' treatment restricts the helpful viability and treatment outcome6-8. Hence, new therapy techniques are direly expected to additionally further develop bosom disease endurance and the life nature of patients.

Fanciful antigen receptor (Vehicle) Lymphocyte treatment is a kind of immunotherapy created from supportive White blood cell movement (ACT)9. In this system, the patient's Lymphocytes are disconnected from autologous fringe blood and further designed ex vivo to communicate engineered receptors that perceive cancer-related antigens (TAAs). Subsequently, Vehicle Immune system microorganisms are refined ex vivo for enhancement and afterward implanted back into patients as an enemy of malignant growth treatment10.

Commonly, Vehicles are made out of four portions

1 A), including an extracellular space for the most part containing a solitary chain variable section

(scFv) got from the variable locale of antibodies for growth antigen acknowledgment, an extracellular spacer directing the distance between Vehicle Lymphocytes and cancer cells, a transmembrane area sticking the manufactured Vehicles to the patient's Immune system microorganism layer, and an intracellular flagging area which comprises CD3ζ and costimulatory areas for Lymphocyte activation9-14. While reaching cancer cells, Vehicle Immune system microorganisms explicitly perceive antigens introduced on the outer layer of growth cells

1B). The clinical aftereffects of the original Vehicle Lymphocyte treatment are unacceptable because the Vehicle White blood cells show unfortunate diligence and fall flat for expansion15-17. To address these issues, Vehicles are additionally designed with costimulatory flagging spaces.

1C). Contrasted and the original of Vehicles, the subsequent age adds one costimulatory area (e.g., CD28, 41BB, ICOS) to the Vehicles to further develop the maintenance period18. The third era of Vehicles further incorporates an additional two costimulatory spaces (e.g., CD27, CD28, 41BB, ICOS, and Bull 40) to improve the constancy and the cytocidal limit of T cells19, 20.

The fourth era of Vehicles, otherwise called Lymphocytes diverted for widespread cytokine-interceded killing [TRUCKs], adds an atomic variable of initiated Immune system microorganisms (NFAT) space holding onto an inducible IL-12 cassette21, 22. In this age, supportive of the fiery cytokine IL-12 is delivered and collected in the designated area after Vehicle White blood cells perceive growth antigens and actuate the downstream flagging pathways. Consequently, the naturally safe cells, including NK cells and macrophages, are selected to grow to tweak the cancer microenvironment and annihilate the disease cells22, 23.

The fifth era of Vehicles is presently under assessment for security and viability, and it is gotten from the second era of Vehicles with an additional IL-2 receptor β-chain section (IL-2Rβ). The IL-2Rβ piece bears a limiting site to set off JAK-Detail flagging pathway enactment. When the Vehicle

Immune system microorganisms target growth antigens, the antigen-explicit enactment of the receptor can set off all the downstream flagging pathways on the double, which brings about Lymphocytes' full actuation and constancy improvement.

Part Five

Intrusive ductal carcinoma

With more than 280,000 individuals analyzed in 2021, bosom disease is the most well-known malignant growth in the US.

The most widely recognized type of bosom malignant growth is intrusive ductal carcinoma (IDC). It's liable for around 70 to 80 percent of all bosom disease analyses.

IDC, otherwise called penetrating ductal carcinoma, gets its name since it starts in the milk-conveying channels of the bosom, and spreads to (or attacks) encompassing bosom tissue.

Obtrusive (or invading) portrays a disease that has spread past its site of beginning. Something contrary to this is "in situ."

Ductal alludes to where IDC begins in the milk conduits. Most bosom tumors start in the conduits or lobules.

Carcinoma alludes to a disease that starts in the skin cells or the tissues coating your interior organs.

Thus, IDC starts and spreads from the milk conduits. This is unmistakable from:

ductal carcinoma in situ (DCIS), which begins in the milk channels but hasn't spread. It's the beginning phase of the disease and may ultimately prompt IDC.

obtrusive lobular carcinoma (ILC), an obtrusive bosom malignant growth that beginnings in the milk-delivering lobules. ILC represents 10% of obtrusive bosom malignant growth analysis. (IDC represents around 80%.)

While IDC can influence individuals at whatever stage in life, it's most often analyzed in ladies ages 55 to 74. This bosom disease can likewise influence men.

What are the side effects of intrusive ductal carcinoma?

You can frequently recognize IDC as a little protuberance in your bosom. However, other potential side effects might be early indications of IDC, including:

expanding of the bosom

thickening of bosom skin

flaky skin on the areola or bosom

skin bothering

peau d'orange

areola withdrawal

areola release, other than bosom milk

diligent bosom or areola torment

Many individuals with IDC experience no side effects. They may not think anything until a specialist tracks down something on a mammogram. Normal screening mammograms can assist with guaranteeing that potential diseases are spotted early.

How is intrusive ductal carcinoma analyzed?

Your PCP might play out a few tests to analyze IDC. Actual test: Your PCP will physically look at your bosom for knots or thickening.

Mammogram: A mammogram is an X-beam of your bosom that can distinguish disease.

Biopsy: Your primary care physician will send an example of your bosom tissue to a lab to be inspected. A bosom biopsy can help decide whether a knot in your bosom is harmful or harmless.

Ultrasound: A bosom ultrasound utilizes sound waves to give an itemized perspective on bosom tissue and bloodstream. It doesn't utilize radiation and is ok for individuals who are pregnant.

X-ray: Attractive reverberation imaging can identify little bosom sores. Specialists use bosom X-rays to screen individuals who have a high gamble of creating bosom disease.

Subtypes of intrusive ductal carcinoma

IDC can show up in more ways than one under a magnifying lens. A biopsy will assist your primary care physician with understanding which subtype of IDC you have.

Around 70% of IDC cases are named with no unique sort (NST). Be that as it may, when the disease cells have unique highlights, they might be named one of the accompanying:

Medullary carcinoma: Another sluggish developing disease, these delicate and meaty cancers look like the medulla of the cerebrum. They represent under 5% of all bosom diseases.

Rounded carcinoma: These are slow-developing growths with disease cells that seem to be tubes. Cylindrical carcinomas represent under 2% of all bosom malignant growths.

Mucinous carcinoma: These second-rate growths contain disease cells that live in mucin, a part of bodily fluid. Mucinous carcinomas represent under 2% of all bosom diseases.

Papillary carcinoma: These are little disease cells with finger-like projections. Papillary carcinomas are interesting, representing under 1% of all bosom diseases.

Cribriform carcinoma: Another intriguing subtype, this disease includes an example of openings that look like Swiss cheddar. They represent under 1% of all bosom diseases.

Metaplastic carcinoma: This happens when ductal cells change structure to become various kinds of cells. Metaplastic carcinomas are typically a more forceful type of malignant growth however represent under 1% of all bosom diseases.

Adenoid cystic carcinoma: These disease cells seem to be malignant growth cells found in the salivary organs than those normally found in ductal cells. They make up under 1% of all bosom malignant growths.

Your bosom disease might be a mix of a portion of the subtypes recorded previously.
HR and HER2 status
How your malignant growth looks under a magnifying lens may not be essentially as significant as a portion of its different highlights. The pathology report from your biopsy will likewise uncover:
chemical receptor (HR) status: whether your disease cells have receptors for the chemicals estrogen and progesterone, which can fuel your disease development

human epidermal development factor receptor 2 (HER2) status: whether your malignant growth cells are delivering excessively (HER2)
Around 80% of bosom tumors are trauma center positive, meaning they test positive for estrogen receptors. Most emergency room-positive bosom diseases are additionally PR-positive, meaning they likewise test positive for progesterone receptors. Something like 2% of malignant growths are PR-positive however emergency room negative.

HER2 proteins exist in sound bosom cells, however, an excessive amount of HER2 can make the disease spread all the more rapidly. Around 14% of bosom tumors are HER2-positive.

You might get a finding of triple-negative bosom malignant growth (TNBC). This implies that your malignant growth isn't delicate to estrogen or progesterone, and you don't have an expanded measure of HER2 protein. TNBC is normally more forceful and will in general have a lower 5-year endurance rate.

Chat with your clinical group to look into what your HR and HER2 status mean for your treatment and standpoint.

How is obtrusive ductal carcinoma organized?

After analysis, the following stage is deciding the phase of your disease. Organizing is a proportion of how enormous your disease has developed and the amount it has spread.

Many elements can impact organizing. Specialists utilize what's called TNM arranging to survey three key variables:

Growth: the size of the essential cancer

Hubs: contribution of adjacent lymph hubs

Metastasis: how much the malignant growth has spread past its essential site.

Consolidating data from those variables, specialists will generally allocate IDC to one of four phases:

Stage 1: a disease that is limited to the bosom with cancer 2 centimeters (cm) or 3/4 inches (in) or less across

Stage 2: a disease that has spread to local lymph hubs in the underarms, or a bosom cancer that is 2 to 5 cm (3/4 to 2 in) across

Stage 3: malignant growth that has spread broadly, however not past the bosom, encompassing tissues, or lymph hubs

Stage 4: disease that has spread to additional far-off locales in the body (metastasized)

DCIS is alluded to as stage 0.

Be that as it may, different elements can likewise impact arranging. They include:

growth grade (how unusual the disease cells look and how rapidly they're probably going to spread)

HR status

HER2 status

These variables can impact treatment and viewpoint.

What causes obtrusive ductal carcinoma?

Bosom malignant growth, including IDC, is brought about by changes to your DNA (transformations). Changes in your bosom cell DNA make the cells develop and separate excessively fast.

The unusual cells bunch together, shaping the knot that you could feel.

Be that as it may, we don't exactly have the foggiest idea of what causes these DNA transformations. Hereditary and natural elements may both assume a part.

What are the gamble factors for intrusive ductal carcinoma?

A few variables increment your gamble of creating bosom malignant growth, including IDC. These include:

Mature: The vast majority are analyzed after the age of 50.

Hereditary qualities: Quality transformations, for example, BRCA1 and BRCA2 changes represent 5 to 10 percent, all things considered.

Family background of bosom or ovarian disease: If a first-degree relative (parent, kin, or kid) or various family members on one side of your family have had bosom or ovarian malignant growth, you're at a higher gamble of creating bosom malignant growth.

Individual history of bosom disease: On the off chance that you've had bosom malignant growth previously, you're three to multiple times as prone to fostering it once more.

Radiation: If you had radiation to your chest to treat an alternate disease before the age of 30, you're at a higher gamble of creating bosom malignant growth.

Regenerative history: Never conveying a youngster to full term or having your most memorable kid after the age of 30 builds your gamble.

Chemical treatment: Long-haul utilization of chemical treatments that incorporate estrogen or progesterone could build your gamble.

Thick bosoms: Ladies with thick bosom tissue are two times as liable to foster malignant growth. Spotting expected diseases on a mammogram is likewise more diligently.

Certain way-of-life factors additionally increment your gamble. They include:
drinking liquor
having stoutness or being overweight

absence of active work

smoking

working around evening time or having high openness to light around evening time

What is the treatment for obtrusive ductal carcinoma?

Assuming you or somebody you realize has been determined to have IDC, have confidence that a wide range of types of treatment are accessible.

The medicines for IDC fall into two fundamental sorts:

Neighborhood therapies for IDC focus on the carcinogenic tissue of the bosom and the encompassing regions, like the chest and lymph hubs. Choices include:

medical procedure

radiation

Fundamental medicines for IDC are applied all through the body, focusing on any cells that might have voyaged and spread from the first cancer.

Foundational therapies are powerful at decreasing the probability that the malignant growth will return after treatment. Choices include:
chemotherapy
hormonal treatment
designated treatment
immunotherapy

Medical procedure

The medical procedure eliminates the harmful growth and decides if the disease has spread to the lymph hubs. The medical procedure is ordinarily the specialist's most memorable reaction while managing IDC. Careful choices include:
lumpectomy, or evacuation of the cancer
mastectomy, or evacuation of the bosom
lymph hub analysis and evacuation

It requires around fourteen days to recuperate from a lumpectomy and a month or more to recuperate from a mastectomy. Recuperation times may be longer assuming you had your lymph hubs eliminated, had remaking done, or on the other hand on the off chance that there were intricacies.

Some of the time your PCP might prescribe non-intrusive treatment to assist with recuperation from this methodology.

Foundational therapies, like chemotherapy, might be given before a medical procedure to contract the growth (neoadjuvant treatment), or after a medical procedure to kill the remaining disease cells (adjuvant treatment).

Radiation

Radiation treatment coordinates strong radiation radiating at the bosom, chest, armpit, or collarbone to kill any cells in or close to the growth area. Radiation treatment requires around 10 minutes to manage every day from 5 to about two months.

Certain individuals treated with radiation might encounter enlarging or skin changes. Certain side effects, like exhaustion, may require 6 to 12 weeks or longer to die down.

Various types of radiation treatments accessible for treating IDC include:

entire bosom radiation, in which outside shaft radiation radiates focus on the whole bosom region

inside halfway bosom radiation, in which radioactive materials are put close to the site of a lumpectomy outer fractional bosom radiation, in which radiation radiates straightforwardly focuses on the first disease site.

Chemotherapy

Chemotherapy comprises anticancer drugs you take in pill structure or utilizing IV. It might require as long as a half year or longer after treatment to recuperate from the many incidental effects, for example, nerve harm, joint torment, and exhaustion.

A wide range of chemotherapy drugs treat ICD, for example, paclitaxel (Taxol) and doxorubicin (Adriamycin). Have a talk with your basic health care doctor about what you want.

Hormonal treatment

Hormonal treatment treats disease cells with receptors for estrogen progesterone, or both. The presence of these chemicals can urge bosom disease cells to increase.

Hormonal treatment eliminates or impedes these chemicals to assist with keeping the malignant growth from developing. Hormonal treatment can have secondary effects that might incorporate hot glimmers and exhaustion.

What amount of time it requires for incidental effects to die down after completing treatment can shift given the medication and the length of the organization.

Some hormonal treatment drugs are taken routinely for a considerable length of time or longer. Secondary effects can require a while to a year or more to wear off whenever treatment has halted.

Sorts of hormonal treatment include:

particular estrogen-receptor reaction modulators, which block the impact of estrogen in the bosom

aromatase inhibitors, which decrease estrogen for postmenopausal ladies

estrogen-receptor down-controllers, which diminish accessible estrogen receptors

ovarian concealment drugs, which briefly prevent ovaries from delivering estrogen

Designated treatments

Designated treatments obliterate bosom disease cells by slowing down unambiguous proteins inside the cell that influence development. Designated treatments can appear as:

monoclonal antibodies, which connect to explicit proteins, such as HER2, to prevent them from developing (e.g., pertuzumab, trastuzumab)

neutralizer drug forms, which join monoclonal antibodies with chemotherapy drugs (e.g., Kadcyla, Enhertu)

kinase inhibitors, which block flags that advise a cell to develop or isolate (e.g., lapatinib, neratinib)

PARP inhibitors, which assist with wiping out cells with transformed BRCA qualities (e.g., olaparib, talazoparib)

Designated treatments are more outlandish than chemotherapy to hurt sound cells, however, they make side impacts. Pregnant ladies shouldn't utilize designated treatments.

Immunotherapy

Your resistant framework doesn't normally recognize malignant growth cells. Immunotherapy drugs assist your resistant framework with spotting disease cells. These include:

designated spot inhibitors, which block the frameworks that hold your safe framework under control (e.g., dostarlimab, pembrolizumab) monoclonal antibodies, which tie to disease cells and permit them to be identified (e.g., pertuzumab, trastuzumab)

Lymphocyte treatment, which permits your Immune system microorganisms to more readily distinguish malignant growth cells (still in clinical preliminaries)

What is the standpoint for intrusive ductal carcinoma?

Your viewpoint on bosom malignant growth relies upon many variables, including

stage at determination

age at analysis

HR and HER2 status

The phase of the malignant growth at analysis means a lot to your standpoint. The 5-year endurance rate for bosom diseases that are as yet limited is no less than 91% for each hormonal subtype.

Assuming that the disease has spread to the lymph hubs or nearby tissue, the 5-year endurance rate ranges somewhere in the range of 65 and 90 percent depending upon the subtype. For a disease that has metastasized, that reach drops to 12 to 38 percent.

With such countless factors, every individual's standpoint is unique. Talk with your clinical group to look into your particular viewpoint in light of variables that are special to you.

Could I at any point forestall obtrusive ductal carcinoma?

Nothing can by and large keep you from creating IDC, however there are sure factors that can bring down your gamble:

keeping a sound weight

remaining genuinely dynamic

keeping away from liquor, or restricting yourself to something like 1 beverage each day

stopping smoking

breastfeeding for quite a long time after labor.

Chemoprevention

If your gamble of getting IDC is high, your primary care physician might endorse drugs that can assist with bringing down your gamble. This is called chemoprevention.

Drugs utilized for chemoprevention include:
tamoxifen (Nolvadex, Soltamox)
raloxifene (Evista)
anastrozole (Arimidex)
exemestane (Aromasin)
However, these medications might have critical side impacts. You and your PCP should gauge the gamble of secondary effects against your gamble of bosom malignant growth.

Action item

Intrusive ductal carcinoma is the most well-known sort of bosom disease. There are neighborhood medicines that target explicit pieces of the body and fundamental treatments that influence the entire body or different organ frameworks.

More than one kind of therapy might be expected to treat bosom disease successfully. Converse with your PCP about the sort of treatment that is appropriate for you.

Part Six

Obtrusive carcinoma

What to Be aware of Intrusive Bosom Malignant growth

Bosom malignant growth, which is the most well-known kind of malignant growth in ladies in the US, is certainly not a solitary sickness. There are, truth be told, a few distinct kinds of bosom disease. One of these is obtrusive bosom disease, in which malignant growth cells spread into encompassing bosom tissues.

This article will carefully describe what obtrusive bosom disease is, how it's analyzed, and the potential treatment choices.

What is intrusive bosom malignant growth?

Bosom malignant growth most frequently starts in the milk-delivering organs (lobules, which are little sacs tracked down inside the curves) or the milk conduits.

At the point when malignant growth cells spread beyond these areas and into solid bosom tissue, it's called intrusive bosom disease.
Most bosom malignant growths are intrusive. As a matter of fact, according to the American Malignant Growth Society, 81% of bosom tumors are an obtrusive sort.

Intrusive bosom malignant growth and organizing
Whether intrusive malignant growth cells are available can impact how bosom disease is organized after a finding.
A bosom disease that stays secluded to the area wherein it began and has not spread into sound bosom tissue is called malignant growth in situ. You may likewise see this alluded to as harmless bosom malignant growth or Stage 0 bosom disease.

At the point when obtrusive malignant growth is distinguished, it very well may be arranged as stages 1 through 4. A considerable lot of these stages likewise have subcategories.
A few variables are thought about with the TNM organizing framework that is utilized for intrusive bosom disease.

Sorts of obtrusive bosom disease

There are various sorts of intrusive bosom diseases. We should look at probably the most widely recognized ones in more detail.

Intrusive ductal carcinoma

Intrusive ductal carcinoma (IDC) is the most widely recognized sort of bosom malignant growth in general. It additionally makes up around 80% of all obtrusive bosom diseases analyzed.

IDC starts in the cells coating the milk conduits. The milk channels are the cylinders in the bosom that convey milk from the lobules to the areola.

In IDC, carcinogenic cells get through the walls of the milk conduit and start to develop into the encompassing bosom tissue. Over the long haul, IDC can spread to lymph hubs and different regions of the body.

Obtrusive lobular carcinoma

Obtrusive lobular carcinoma (ILC) is the second most normal kind of intrusive bosom disease. Around 10% of intrusive bosom diseases are ILC.

Obtrusive lobular carcinoma starts in the lobules, which are the organs in the bosom that make milk. In ILC, disease cells have gotten through the mass of the lobule and into adjoining bosom tissue. Like intrusive ductal carcinoma, ILC can likewise spread to different regions of the body.

Because of the way that it develops, ILC can at times be more enthusiastically identified through screening techniques like a bosom test or mammogram. It's likewise conceivable that around 1 out of 5 ladies with ILC can have malignant growth that influences the two bosoms.

More uncommon sorts

Different kinds of intrusive bosom malignant growth are more uncommon. These can incorporate fiery bosom disease and triple-negative bosom malignant growth.

Also, obtrusive ductal carcinoma has a few subtypes that, together, make up less than 5% of all bosom malignant growths. These are depicted because of how they look under a magnifying lens and include:

adenoid cystic carcinoma

medullary carcinoma

metaplastic carcinoma

micropapillary carcinoma

blended carcinoma

mucinous carcinoma
papillary carcinoma
rounded carcinoma

What are the side effects?

It's conceivable that intrusive bosom malignant growth might not have any perceptible side effects. In these cases, it could be at first distinguished through routine screening procedures like a mammogram.

Available side effects can include:
another irregularity or thickening that can be felt in the bosom or underarm (armpit) region
Swap in the bigness or state of the breast
skin changes on the breast, like redness, expanding or dimpling
an areola that turns internal
liquid that breaks from the areola that is not breastmilk.

How could it be analyzed?

There are different tests to analyze obtrusive bosom malignant growth. These include:

Bosom test: During a bosom test, a medical services professional will cautiously feel your bosoms for indications of protuberances or different changes.

Mammogram: During a mammogram, a gadget presses your bosoms between two plates. X-beam pictures of the bosom tissue are then taken and assessed for indications of disease.

Imaging tests: A medical service proficient may arrange extra imaging tests to assist them with better-picturing bosom tissue. A few models incorporate ultrasound or attractive reverberation imaging (X-ray).

Biopsy: During a biopsy, an example of bosom tissue is painstakingly taken out and looked at under a magnifying lens for indications of malignant growth.

Blood tests: Blood tests utilize an example your blood to check for different markers of infection or sickness.

Assuming the disease is identified, extra tests can be utilized to assist with portraying the malignant growth and decide its stage. These tests can incorporate things like:

Receptor testing: Different tests can check for estrogen receptors, progesterone receptors, and HER2 status.

Lymph hub biopsy: A lymph hub biopsy can decide whether the malignant growth has spread to the close by lymph hubs.

Imaging tests: Imaging tests can hope to check whether malignant growth has spread to different regions. Some that might be utilized incorporate bone sweeps, X-beams, CT outputs, and positron discharge tomography (PET) checks.

How is intrusive bosom malignant growth ordinarily treated?

Therapy for intrusive bosom malignant growth relies upon the phase of the disease as well as different variables. We should inspect the most widely recognized treatment choices.

Medical procedure

Numerous ladies have a medical procedure to eliminate the malignant growth cells and the lymph hubs that the disease has spread to. The kind of medical procedure suggested relies upon the disease stage, as well as the area of the cancer.

Sorts of a medical procedure

Bosom saving a medical procedure: Bosom preserving a medical procedure eliminates the cancer and a portion of the encompassing tissue, however, it doesn't include expulsion of the bosom. It's likewise called a halfway mastectomy or a lumpectomy.

Complete mastectomy: An all-out mastectomy eliminates the whole bosom. It might likewise eliminate a portion of the lymph hubs that are found near the armpit.

Changed revolutionary mastectomy: A changed extremist mastectomy eliminates the whole bosom, a significant number of the encompassing lymph hubs, and probably the chest lining. Some of the time a piece of the chest muscle is eliminated too.

Radiation treatment

Radiation treatment utilizes high-energy radiation to prevent malignant growth cells from developing. It can either be given remotely or inside (brachytherapy).

Radiation treatment is often suggested after a medical procedure. That is because it can help dispose of any disease cells that might have stayed behind at the careful site.

Foundational treatments

Foundational treatments will be medicines that can go through your circulation system, influencing various pieces of your body.

Foundational treatments can be given as a pill or implantation.

Instances of foundational treatments include:

Chemotherapy: Chemotherapy comprises areas of strength for of that can keep malignant growth cells from developing.

Choose a treatment: choose treatment that utilizes drugs that specifically kill disease cells. Along these lines, they hurt solid cells in the body contrasted with chemotherapy and radiation treatment.

Chemical treatment: Chemical treatment hinders the activities of chemicals that can make bosom disease cells develop. It very well may be utilized on the off

chance that bosom disease is positive for particular kinds of chemical receptors, like estrogen or progesterone.

Immunotherapy: Immunotherapy works by animating invulnerable cells to answer disease cells. Treating a few kinds of intrusive bosom disease, for example, triple-negative bosom cancer can be utilized.

Foundational treatments might be prescribed before a medical procedure to assist with contracting a growth, especially on the off chance that the cancer is enormous. This is called neoadjuvant treatment.
Like radiation treatment, these therapies can likewise be utilized after a medical procedure, to assist with eliminating any excess disease cells that might in any case be available at the careful site.

This is called adjuvant treatment.
Since foundational treatments can go all through the body, they're likewise the primary therapy choice for

individuals who have metastatic bosom malignant growth.

What's the contrast between obtrusive and metastatic bosom malignant growth?

Obtrusive bosom malignant growth essentially alludes to bosom disease that has spread away from the tissue wherein it began and into sound bosom tissue. It very well may be either limited or metastatic.

For instance, assuming a malignant growth that starts in the milk channels gets through the covering of the milk pipes and spreads into solid bosom tissue, that disease is viewed as obtrusive. Nonetheless, it's not metastatic because it's confined to the bosom.

Assuming that disease cells split away from that growth and spread to different regions of the body, for example, the liver or lungs, the disease is currently metastatic. For this situation, the bosom disease is both obtrusive and metastatic.

What's the anticipation for intrusive bosom disease?

Overall, they are as yet alive 5 years after their finding.

As indicated by the American Malignant Growth Society, the 5-year endurance rates for the bosom disease are resolved in light of how far the malignant growth has spread at the hour of determination.

For example: 5-year endurance rates for bosom disease

Confined: When bosom malignant growth stays limited to the bosom, the 5-year endurance is close to 100%.

Provincial: Assuming that bosom disease has spread to lymph hubs or adjoining tissues, the 5-year endurance rate is 86%.

Far off: Assuming bosom disease has spread to additional far-off tissues of the body (metastasized), the 5-year endurance rate is 28%.

In general: The general 5-year endurance rate for bosom disease is 90%.

It's memorable's vital that these numbers are obtained from an extraordinary number of individuals determined to have bosom disease. While these numbers can be useful, they can't anticipate what will befall you.

Each individual is unique. While factors like stage and attributes of the disease positively influence viewpoint, individual elements like age and generally speaking well-being are additionally significant. Also, fresher, more compelling therapies keep on being created, which works on the anticipation for bosom disease.

Bosom malignant growth support

The physical, mental, and profound cost of bosom malignant growth can at times feel overpowering. While this is typical, there are numerous assets accessible to help, including the following:

The Bosom Disease Healthline application puts a local area of help right readily available. Utilizing the Healthline application, you can associate with different individuals who have comparative interests, treatment plans, and inquiries to your own. Download it here.

The American Disease Society gives various administrations, including an all-day, every-day helpline (800-227-2345), associations with bosom malignant growth survivors, and transportation to treatment focuses.

Breastcancer.org gives data about bosom disease, therapy choices, and everyday subjects like nourishment and exercise. Its conversation sheets and web recording can assist you with associating with others who've been determined to have bosom malignant growth.

Living Past Bosom Malignant Growth (LBBC) is committed to offering help administrations to individuals living with bosom disease, bosom malignant growth survivors, and friends and family. You can associate with others face to face, on the web, or by telephone.

The Communities for Infectious Prevention and Avoidance (CDC) can assist you with tracking down minimal expense screenings. Furthermore, it likewise offers web recordings and recordings on an assortment of bosom disease subjects.

Part Seven

Bosom malignant growth research establishment

Bosom Malignant Growth Exploration Establishment

The Bosom Malignant Growth Exploration Establishment (BCRF) is a not-for-profit focused on counteraction methodologies and accomplishing a remedy for bosom disease. BCRF gives financing to disease research overall to fuel propels in cancer science, hereditary qualities, counteraction, therapy, metastasis, and survivorship.

As indicated by Good Cause Pilot, BCRF puts around 87% of its assets toward projects and administrations and under 4% is spent on authoritative expenses.

Bosom Malignant growth Secret stash

The Bosom Malignant Growth Rainy Day account is an association situated in the San Francisco Straight Region. They're committed to giving crisis monetary help to low-pay ladies and men with bosom disease. The asset gifts the vast majority of its assortments — 59% — to people, yet evenly divides the rest:

15% goes to bosom disease establishments

22% is given to bosom malignant growth associations

4% is reinvested in the asset.

The Rose

The Rose is the main not-for-profit bosom medical services association in southeast Texas. Its board ensured radiologists, specific specialized staff, two mammography, and indicative imaging habitats, and an armada of portable mammography vans offer high-level bosom disease screening, demonstrative administrations, and admittance to treatment to more than 40,000 ladies every year.

Since its send-off in 1986, The Rose has offered types of assistance to a portion of 1,000,000 ladies.

SHARE Malignant growth Backing

SHARE is a public charity that backs, instructs, and engages ladies impacted by bosom or ovarian malignant growth. It puts an extraordinary spotlight on therapeutically underserved networks. Its central goal is to make and support a strong local area of ladies impacted by bosom or ovarian disease.

Offer's administrations are all for nothing and they incorporate care groups, instructive apparatuses, and clinical preliminary help.

Breastcancer.org

The mission of Breastcancer.org is to give the most solid, complete, and exceptional data about bosom disease.

This charitable hopes to help those determined to have the infection and their friends and family gain a superior comprehension of bosom well-being and bosom malignant growth on a clinical and individual level.

Dana-Farber Malignant Growth Organization

However the Dana-Farber Disease Establishment in Boston, Massachusetts centers around different kinds of malignant growth, they truly do run a particular program that works with people who have gotten a bosom disease determination.

The Susan F. Smith Place for Ladies' Tumors at Dana-Farber offers those with bosom malignant growth different therapy choices, which incorporate "the most recent clinical oncology and careful choices," notwithstanding bosom reproduction and radiation treatment.

CancerCare

CancerCare, established in 1944, expects to assist people adapting to various difficulties related to bosom malignant growth — close to home, down to earth, and monetary — by offering free proficient help administrations and data.

CancerCare reports that they've given $76.4 million in monetary help to almost 31,000 individuals to

assist with therapy-related expenses, for example, transportation, home consideration, kid care, and co-installment help.

Bosom disease support administrations

Around 1 in every 8 U.S. individuals brought into the world of the female sex will foster bosom malignant growth in the course of their lives. Living with and dealing with this illness can incur significant damage.

Good cause — both at the neighborhood and public levels — gives required assets to people and families impacted by bosom disease, while offering administrations like care groups, monetary help, and direction on treatment choices.

Conclusion

Bosom malignant growth is a sickness where cells in the bosom outgrow control. It is caused by changes in the hereditary material (DNA) and can spread externally to the bosom through veins and lymph vessels. The most common types of bosom disease are obtrusive ductal carcinoma, lobular carcinoma, Paget illness of the bosom, phyllodes growth, and angiosarcoma. It can spread externally to the bosom through veins and lymph vessels and metastasize to different pieces of the body. It can be prevented by making solid way-of-life changes such as staying at a solid weight, restricting liquor use, getting enough exercise, restricting openness to estrogen by breastfeeding infants if possible, and restricting chemical treatment. It is important to get regular mammograms to detect bosom malignant growth in the beginning phases when it is more straightforward to treat.

Ductal carcinoma in situ (DCIS) is an early bosom disease that involves the presence of strange cells inside a milk conduit in the bosom. It is viewed as the earliest type of bosom malignant growth and

requires an assessment and a thought of treatment choices. Risk elements include expanding age, the individual history of harmless bosom infection, family background of bosom disease, never having been pregnant, Having your most memorable child after the age of 30, Having your most memorable period before age 12, Starting menopause after age 55, hereditary changes that increment the gamble of bosom malignant growth, like those in the bosom disease qualities BRCA1 and BRCA2. Treatment for DCIS relies on every lady's circumstance. More often than before, specialists can offer moderate treatment. Radiation treatment can have side impacts, and there is no proof of any advantage from axillary analyzation in ladies with DCIS 1. For certain ladies, the specialist will suggest a mastectomy (evacuation of the impacted bosom).
Ductal bosom malignant growth is the most common type of bosom disease in the US, with around 297,790 individuals in the US expected to have a bosom malignant growth finding in 2023.

There are two types of ductal bosom disease: obtrusive ductal carcinoma (IDC) and ductal carcinoma in situ (DCIS). Risk factors for ductal bosom malignant growth include progress in years,

liquor use, certain conceptive elements, thick bosom tissue, family background of bosom disease, qualities, history of bosom disease, chemical treatment, smoking tobacco, and postmenopausal estrogen and progesterone prescriptions. To identify ductal bosom malignant growth, a medical care professional will physically analyze the bosom for protuberances or thickening, perform a mammogram, biopsy, ultrasound, attractive reverberation imaging (X-ray), and attractive reverberation imaging (X-ray) to screen individuals with a high gamble of creating bosom disease.

Ductal bosom malignant growth (DCIS) is an uncommon condition where strange cells are fostered in the milk organs, known as lobules, in the bosom. LCIS is an uncommon condition where strange cells are held inside the inward covering of the lobules and require no treatment past careful evacuation. LCIS is a treatable condition and the viewpoint is great for the individuals who are determined to have it. LCIS is usually analyzed on a bosom biopsy performed for a strange mammogram and is usually seen on a minute assessment of the bosom tissue. Bosom excisional biopsy is a minor strategy performed by a specialist to eliminate a

the somewhat bigger measure of bosom tissue where LCIS was distinguished. The 5-year relative endurance rate for DCIS is around 90.8%, with limited bosom malignant growth having a 99.3% 5-year relative endurance rate and regionalized bosom disease having an 86.3% 5-year relative endurance rate. LCIS is a treatable condition and the viewpoint is great for the individuals who are determined to have it.

Lobular Carcinoma in Situ (LCIS) is the most commonly analyzed malignant growth around the world, with 2.3 million new cases and 685,000 patient passings in 2020. Vehicle Immune System Microorganism Treatment (Vehicle) Lymphocyte treatment is a sort of immunotherapy created from supportive White blood cell movement, which ordinarily utilizes patients' insusceptible cells to battle disease. This survey aims to examine the advancement of Vehicle White blood cell treatment in bosom disease from preclinical examinations to continuous clinical preliminaries. The global disease measurements in 2020 show bosom malignant growth have superseded cellular breakdown in the lungs and become the most normally analyzed malignant growth around the world, with 2.3 million

new cases in 11.7% of all disease types reported. The histological characterization of bosom disease is based on the articulation example of human epidermal development factor receptors 2 (HER2) and chemical receptors (HR) named estrogen receptors (emergency room) and progesterone receptors (PR), as well as the growth expansion rate shown.

Fanciful antigen receptor (Vehicle) Lymphocyte treatment is a kind of immunotherapy created from supportive White blood cell movement (ACT). It involves the patient's Lymphocytes being disconnected from autologous fringe blood and further designed ex vivo to communicate engineered receptors that perceive cancer-related antigens (TAAs). Vehicles are made out of four portions, including an extracellular spacer directing the distance between Vehicle Lymphocytes and cancer cells, a transmembrane area sticking the manufactured Vehicles to the patient's Immune system microorganism layer, and an intracellular flagging area which comprises CD3 and costimulatory areas for Lymphocyte activation. To address these issues, Vehicles are also designed with costimulatory flagging spaces. The fifth era of

Vehicles are presently under assessment for security and viability, and it is gotten from the second era of Vehicles with an additional IL-2 receptor-chain section (IL-2R).

Adenoid cystic carcinoma (IDC) is a malignant growth found in the salivary organs of the bosom. It is organized into four phases: Stage 1, Stage 2, Stage 3, and Stage 4. It is caused by changes to the DNA (transformations) in the bosom cell DNA, which make the cells develop and separate excessively fast. Gamble factors for IDC include age, hereditary qualities, family background, individual history of bosom or ovarian disease, radiation, regenerative history, chemical treatment, thick bosoms, smoking, working around evening time or having high openness to light around evening time, and certain way-of-life factors. Treatment for IDC includes chemotherapy, hormonal treatment, designated treatment, immunotherapy, and radiotherapy.

The most important details in this text are the medical procedures used to treat intrusive ductal carcinoma (IDC). The medical procedure involves eliminating the harmful growth and determining if the disease has spread to the lymph hubs. Radiation treatment involves strong radiation radiating at the

bosom, chest, armpit, or collarbone to kill any cells in or close to the growth area. Chemotherapy comprises anticancer drugs that take in pill structure or utilizing IV. Hormonal treatment treats disease cells with receptors for estrogen progesterone, or both. Designated treatments obliterate bosom disease cells by slowing down unambiguous proteins inside the cell that influence development. Immunotherapy drugs assist the resistant framework with spotting disease cells. The 5-year endurance rate for bosom diseases that are as yet limited is no less than 91% for each hormonal subtype. The 5-year endurance rate ranges somewhere in the range of 65 and 90 percent depending upon the subtype. The 5-year survival rate for IDC that has metastasized is 12 to 38 percent. The 5-year survival rate for IDC that has metastasized is 12 to 38 percent.

Obtrusive bosom malignant growth is the most common kind of malignant growth in ladies in the US, with 81% of bosom tumors being an obtrusive sort. There are various types of obtrusive bosom diseases, such as intrusive ductal carcinoma (IDC), obtrusive lobular carcinoma (ILC), fiery bosom disease, and triple-negative bosom malignant

growth. The most common symptoms of intrusive bosom malignant growth include irregularities or thickening in the bosom or underarm (armpit) region, skin changes on the breast, and changes in the size or state of the breast.

The most important details in this text are the types of medical procedures used to treat bosom malignant growth. These include a medical procedure called a halfway mastectomy or lumpectomy, a complete mastectomy, a changed revolutionary mastectomy, radiation treatment, foundational treatments, neoadjuvant treatment, and adjuvant treatment. Foundational treatments include chemotherapy, choose treatment, chemical treatment, immunotherapy, and neoadjuvant treatment. Obtrusive bosom malignant growth has a 5-year endurance rate of 90%, while metastatic bosom malignant growth has a 5-year endurance rate of 90%. Support services such as the Bosom Disease Healthline application, the American Disease Society, Breastcancer.org, Living Past Bosom

Malignant Growth (LBBC), and the Communities for Infectious Prevention and Avoidance (CDC) are available to help individuals living with bosom malignant growth.

The Bosom Malignant Growth Exploration Establishment (BCRF) is a not-for-profit focused on counteraction methodologies and accomplishing a remedy for bosom disease. It gives financing to disease research overall to fuel propels in cancer science, hereditary qualities, counteraction, therapy, metastasis, and survivorship. The Bosom Malignant Growth Rainy Day account is an association situated in the San Francisco Straight Region that gives crisis monetary help to low-pay ladies and men with bosom disease. SHARE is a public charity that backs, instructs, and engages ladies impacted by bosom or ovarian malignant growth. Breastcancer.org provides the most solid, complete, and exceptional data about bosom disease. Dana-Farber Malignant Growth Organization offers people with bosom malignant growth different therapy choices. CancerCare provides free proficient help administrations and data to assist people adapting to various difficulties related to bosom malignant growth.